YOUR KNOWLEDGE HAS VALUE

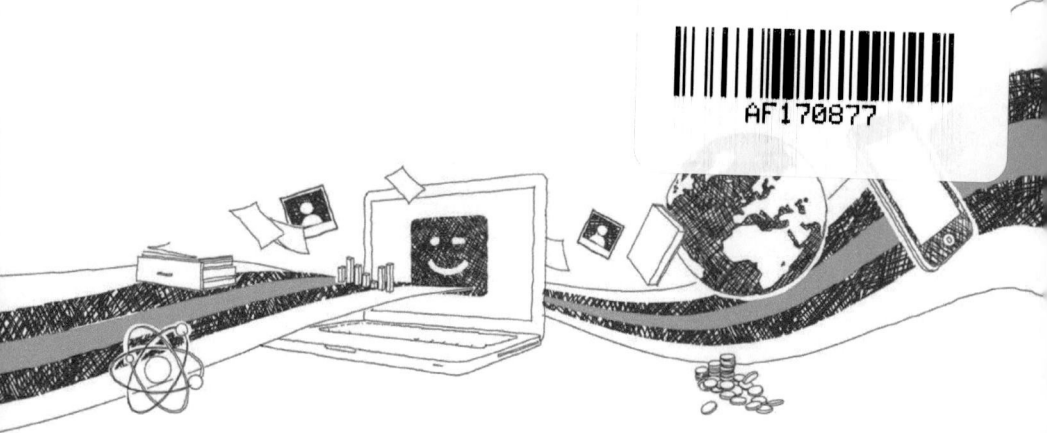

- We will publish your bachelor's and master's thesis, essays and papers

- Your own eBook and book - sold worldwide in all relevant shops

- Earn money with each sale

Upload your text at www.GRIN.com and publish for free

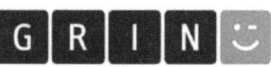

Bibliographic information published by the German National Library:

The German National Library lists this publication in the National Bibliography; detailed bibliographic data are available on the Internet at http://dnb.dnb.de .

This book is copyright material and must not be copied, reproduced, transferred, distributed, leased, licensed or publicly performed or used in any way except as specifically permitted in writing by the publishers, as allowed under the terms and conditions under which it was purchased or as strictly permitted by applicable copyright law. Any unauthorized distribution or use of this text may be a direct infringement of the author s and publisher s rights and those responsible may be liable in law accordingly.

Imprint:

Copyright © 2015 GRIN Verlag
Print and binding: Books on Demand GmbH, Norderstedt Germany
ISBN: 9783668865679

This book at GRIN:

https://www.grin.com/document/452520

Mitiku Wamile

Retrospective Analysis of Suspected Rabies Cases in Lemu-Bilbilo District, Arsi Zone, Ethiopia

GRIN Verlag

GRIN - Your knowledge has value

Since its foundation in 1998, GRIN has specialized in publishing academic texts by students, college teachers and other academics as e-book and printed book. The website www.grin.com is an ideal platform for presenting term papers, final papers, scientific essays, dissertations and specialist books.

Visit us on the internet:

http://www.grin.com/

http://www.facebook.com/grincom

http://www.twitter.com/grin_com

RETROSPECTIVE ANALYSIS OF SUSPECTED RABIES CASES IN LEMU-BILBILO DISTRICT, ARSI ZONE, ETHIOPIA

BY:
MITIKU WAMILE

A THESIS SUBMITTED TO COLLEGE OF VETERINARY MEDICINE AND AGRICULTURE, ADDISABABA UNIVERSITY IN PARTIAL FULFILMENT OF REQUIREMENT FOR ATTAINMENT OF DEGREE, DOCTOR OF VETERINARY MEDICINE (DVM)

JUNE, 2015
BISHOFTU, ETHIOPIA

TABLE OF CONTENTS	Pages
ACKNOWLEDGEMENTS	I
LIST OF ABBREVIATIONS	II
LIST OF TABLES	III
LIST OF FIGURES	IV
ABSTRACT	V
1. INTRODUCTION	1
2. MATERIALS AND METHODS	4
2.1. Description of the Study Area	4
2.2. Study Design	4
3. ETHICAL ISSUES	5
4. DATA MANAGEMENT AND ANALYSIS	5
5. RESULT	6
5.1. Bite incidence	6
5.2. Age and Gender of the Victim	6
5.3. Seasonal distribution of bites	7
5.4. Type of biting animal	8
5.5. Status of dogs involved in the bite	8
5.6. Ownership of biting animals	9
5.7. Anatomical site of bite	10
5.8. Severity of bite	10
5.9. Rabies post exposure prophylaxis and wound management	11
5.10. Severity and anatomic locations of bite wound	11
5.11. D Distribution of bite injuries on the body according to age group of dog bite patients	12
6. DISCUSSION	13
7. CONCLUSION AND RECOMMENDATIONS	16
8. REFERENCES	17

ACKNOWLEDGEMENTS

First of all, I would like to thanks GOD almighty who has been giving me everything: Patience, health, wisdom, and blessing. I give Him the Honor and Glory, for His all time goodwill and assistance in general, for giving me the courage and endurance to start the studies and finalize this thesis in particular.

I would like to gratefully and sincerely thank Dr. Tariku Jibat for his guidance, understanding, patience, encouragement throughout this work and devotion of his time in correcting this thesis and most importantly, his friendship during my studies

Also I deeply express my heartfelt special thanks for all my classmates for their social life contributions during preceding six year. I will never forget my entire close friend during my academic years here, Biyansa, Gamachu, Itafa, Lama, Matios(Monenus),Motuma,, Olana, Tefera, and to all friends that I can't mention here. I will not forget everything that we've shared together.

Finally, I am also grateful to my mom, my sisters and my brothers for their love and encouragements; for providing me with unfailing support and continuous encouragement throughout my years of life. This accomplishment would not have been possible without them.

LIST OF ABBREVIATIONS

CSA	Central Statistics Agency
DALYs	Disability Adjusted Life Years
masl	mean above sea level
PEP	Post Exposure Prophylaxis
SPSS	Statistical Package for Social Sciences
WHO	World Health Organization

LIST OF TABLES **Pages**

Table 1: Age and gender distribution of dog bites..7
Table 2: Species of biting animal..8
Table 3: Status of biting animals...9
Table 4: Rabies post exposure prophylaxis and other practices...11
Table 5: Distribution of bite injuries on the body according to age group 12

LIST OF FIGURES   **Pages**

Figure 1: Age distribution of victims..6

Figure 2: Seasonal distribution of bite victims..7

Figure 3: Ownership of biting animal...9

Figure 4: anatomic location of dog bite wounds of the victim..10

Figure 5: shows wound severity..10

Figure 6: Comparison of age class and body part bitten..12

ABSTRACT

This study aimed to estimate the incidence of human dog bites, describe characteristics of bites and to identify risk factors for dog bites in Lemu-Bilbilo district. A retrospective analysis of suspected rabies cases (dog bites) in Lemu- Bilbilo district during the period 2013/2014 ($n=1$ year) was done. A total of 316 bite injuries inflicted by rabies-suspected animals were reported, giving a mean annual incidence of ~137 cases per 100,000. Males (56.6%) were more at risk than females (43.4%). The proportion of children (0-19 aged) bitten was relatively higher than that of adults. 34.2% of victims were bitten by neighbour dogs. Domestic dogs were involved in 95% of the human bite cases, whereas man (1.9%), donkey (1.6%), cattle (0.9%), wild animal (0.3%) and horse (0.3%) played a minor role. 94.3 % of the victims mentioned that the disease (rabies) status of the dogs involved in the bite incidents was rabid. Rabies-suspected case reports were most frequently occurred during August and October in each year. This study revealed that incidences of humans being bitten by dogs suspected of rabies are common in Lemu-Bilbilo, involve mostly children and predominantly occur during autumn. Rigorous surveillance to determine the status of rabies and the risk factors for human rabies, and increased educational awareness of people about the risk of dog bites and rabies at national level is necessary, particularly for children as well as formulation and institution of appropriate rabies-control policies, is required.

Key words: *Ethiopia, Human animal bites, Lemu-Bilbilo, Oromia, Rabies*

1. INTRODUCTION

Rabies is a highly fatal, zoonotic disease that causes severe destruction of the central nervous system of all warm-blooded animals. Typically, humans acquire rabies following the bite of a rabid animal. Domestic dogs (*Canisfamiliaris*) play a key role in the transmission of rabies to humans (WHO, 2001).

Rabies is endemic in developing countries of Africa and Asia, and most human deaths from the disease occur in these endemic countries (WHO, 1998). The vast majority (99%) of human deaths arising from rabies occur in the tropical developing world. About 24,000 to 70,000 people are estimated to die of rabies each year in Africa and Asia (WHO, 1998; Warrell, D. and Warell, M. 1995). Human mortality from endemic canine rabies was estimated to be 55, 000 deaths per year and was responsible for 1.74 million disability adjusted life years (DALYs) losses each year. The annual cost of rabies in Africa and Asia was estimated at US$ 583.5 million most of which is due to cost of post exposure prophylaxis (PEP) (Knobel *et al.*, 2005).

Ethiopia being one of the developing countries is highly endemic for rabies. Approximately 10, 000 people were estimated to die of rabies annually in Ethiopia which makes it to be one of the worst affected countries in the world (Fekadu *et al.*, 1997). Most of the incidences of human rabies occur in rural areas. It has been proposed that this is due to a number of reasons, including low vaccination coverage of dogs as a result of inadequate awareness of the problem, as well as inability to finance the costs of vaccination; poor management of dogs, in particular the free movement of dogs, which increases their risk of contracting rabies from wildlife (Knobel *et al.*, 2005) and although effective and economical control measures are available, rabies remains a neglected disease in terms of policy formulations throughout most of the developing countries (Bogel and Meslin, 1990; Cleaveland *et al.*, 2003).

In Ethiopia individuals who are exposed to rabies virus often see traditional healers for the diagnosis and treatment of the disease (Deressa *et al.*, 2010). These widespread traditional practices of handling rabies cases are believed to interfere with timely seeking of PEP. Rabies victims especially from rural areas seek PEP treatment after exhausting the traditional medicinal intervention and usually after a loss of life from family members (Deressa et al., 2010).

Dogs are the principal source of infection for humans and livestock (Deressa et al., 2010). In Ethiopia many households own dogs usually for guarding property. Although there are no formal studies, it is estimated that there is one owned dog per five household nationally. Dog management is often poor and dog vaccination is limited to few dogs in urban centers. High population of dogs with poor management contributes for high endemicity of canine rabies in Ethiopia. In canine rabies endemic countries like Ethiopia, rabies has also significant economic importance by its effect on livestock (Deressa et al., 2010).

Dog bites are a significant cause of morbidity and mortality worldwide, particularly where rabies is endemic. There has been steady increase in the incidence of dog bites; rabies transmission. Controlling rabies in urban dog populations is seen as a more cost-effective, long-term way to prevent human rabies than reliance on post exposure human treatment (Bogel and Meslin, 1990). In most developed countries several large areas have successfully eliminated canine rabies through legislation, education, and mass vaccination of dog. Cities in poorer countries such as Ethiopia, however, lag behind in control efforts due to various socioeconomic factors and low understanding of the actual trend of the disease. To achieve control, knowledge of the epidemiology of rabies in dog populations has long been recognized as crucial (WHO, 1987).This will be crucial for effective planning of rabies management, prevention or control programs. Throughout the world, it has been found that children are more at risk of getting bitten by dogs. Animal bites might also serve as an important route of transmission for a number of diseases, most importantly rabies, which still remains endemic in large parts of the world. The World Health Organisation states that 99% of all human rabies cases are caused by infected dog saliva (WHO, 2013).

If used keenly, reports of animal-bite injuries would aid in estimating area or region-specific disease burden, thus enabling giving priority to improved rabies surveillance and control. Reports of animal-bite victims in the hospitals and health centers are examples of resources for such information. Such reports would assist in identifying characteristics of patients reporting (age, sex); areas with frequent incidences of animal bites; species of animals involved and period with high incidence of bite injuries. These insights would prompt surveillance providers to better understand how dog population size, movements, accessibility and habitat affect the transmission of rabies. There is also a significant financial burden attached to prophylactic treatment to diminish the risk of rabies infection (Humphrey *et al.*, 2010).

Analysis of retrospective data and current information on rabies in humans with special focus is important to understand the epidemiological situation of rabies. Epidemiological studies provide basic information about the burden of the disease and underline the importance of prevention and control interventions. But, there is lack of accurate quantitative information on rabies both in humans and animals and little is known about the awareness of the people about the disease to apply effective control measures in Ethiopia. There have been also limited studies conducted regarding the incidence of rabies and associated risk factors and over the years; cases of dog bites are on the increase which necessitated the desire to evaluate the status of the problem in Ethiopia. The objectives of the study were; therefore, to estimate the incidence of human dog bites, describe characteristics of bites and to identify risk factors for dog bites in Lemu-Bilbilo district

2. MATERIALS AND METHODS

2.1. Description of the study area

The study was conducted in Lemu-Bilbilo district located in Arsi zone; Oromia Regional State of Ethiopia. Lemu-Bilbilo is located at 7°31'60" N latitude and 39°15'0" E longitude. It is characterized by a crop-livestock mixed farming system. It is located at an elevation of 2,809 masl. Lemu-Bilbilo district is located about 235km South-east of the capital Addis Ababa on the highway towards Bale zone. The area receives an annual rainfall of 1100 mm, of which more than 85% is during the main rainy season (June to November).The 2013/14 national census reported a total population of urban and rural residence for this woreda was 231,795, of whom 114,149 were men and 117,646 were women(CSA,2014).

2.2. Study design

About the epidemiology of dog bite and bite-victim's knowledge about rabies, detailed list of suspected rabid dog victims were collected from health centers and then these lists were given to health extension workers in each village. These health extension workers contacted all victims in the village visited health centers, traditional healers and even those who went nowhere for the period of one year from September 11, 2013 until September 10, 2014. These victims were interviewed using a pre-tested structured questionnaire designed to obtain information on the bite and its circumstances, and the biting animal.

The survey was conducted from 30 November 2014 to 8 February 2015. The information gathered included, address of victims, date of attendance, sex, age, bite time season, site of the bite injury, severity of wound, type of treatment given, origin of biting animal, traditional treatment, species of the animal that bit them ,ownership of biting animals.

3. ETHICAL ISSUES

The study was ethically approved by Oromia-Regional-Health-Bureau (ORHB)

4. DATA MANAGEMENT AND ANALYSIS

The data collected were entered into Microsoft Office Excel 2007. The data were checked for their completeness and consistency; duplicates and those incomplete and inconsistent were corrected when possible and removed otherwise. Description of the results from the cleaned data was done by descriptive statistics and chi square for comparison. The estimated incidence of the disease in humans was calculated by dividing bite victims and probable rabies cases by the population at risk. The incidence estimates were expressed as cases per 100, 000 individuals at risk per year

The data collected was subjected to statistical package for social sciences (SPSS) version 21 for analysis. Descriptive statistics was used to analyse the rate, frequency and proportions. Chi-square tests were used to compare the difference in proportions of dog bites between gender, age group and other variables.

5. RESULT

A total of 319 patients were interviewed. Three questionnaires were excluded from the analyses because they were suspected to be duplicates. The final analysis was undertaken on 316 dog bite questionnaires,

5.1. Bite incidence

During the 1-year period (2013/2014), a total of 316 bite injuries by rabies-suspected animals were recorded at Lemu-Bilbilo district, giving a mean annual incidence of ~137 cases per 100,000 (56.6% males, 43.4% females).

5.2. Age and gender of the victim:

This study shows males comprised 56.6% of the cases, and 55.4% of the total were under 20 years old. However, those in the age groups 0-29 years were the most common victims of dog bites with the number decreasing thereafter with age (figure 1).There were significantly more bite cases in males than females. This study showed that the incidence of dog bites was greater amongst children aged 0–19.9 years and greater in males than females across all age groups (Table 1.).

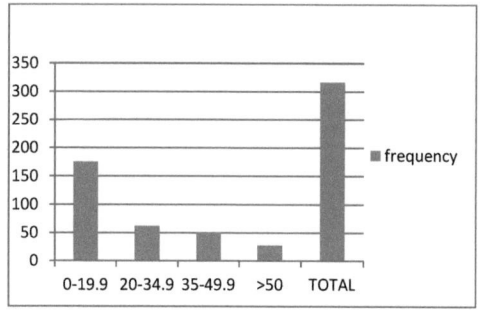

Figure 1 .Age distributions of victim

Table 1: age and gender distribution of dog bites

		Age				Total
		0-19.9	20-34.5	35-49.9	Above 50	
Sex	Male	93(29.4%)	37(11.7%)	31(9.8%)	18(5.69%)	**179(56.6%)**
	Female	82(25.9%)	25(7.9%)	20(6.3%	10(5.69%)	**137(43.4)**
Total		**175(55.3%)**	**62(19.6%)**	**51(1.1%)**	**28(8.8%)**	**316(100%)**

5.3. Seasonal distribution of bites

Dog bite incidents were reported throughout the year with more bite incidents during the summer month (June -august (80/316; 25.3%) followed by winter (December -February) (63/316; 19.9%) and autumn month (September -November) (61/316; 19.4%) and the reported incidents were lowest during the spring month (March -may) (41/316; 12.9%) (Figure 2).

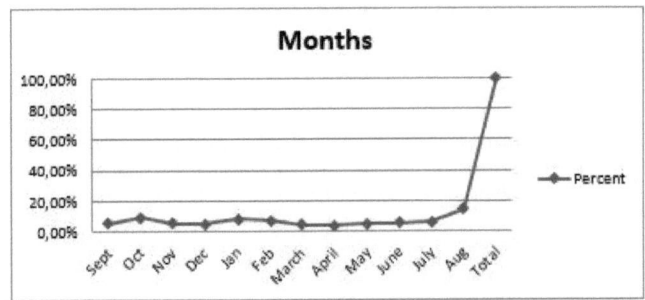

Figure 2: Seasonal distribution of bite victims

5.4. Type of biting Animal:

Among bites by various animals, dog bites being the major (95%) cause of injury to humans. Human bites by species other than dogs were also reported. The other species included Cattle, wild animals (hyena and foxes), horse, Donkey and man.

Table 2: Species of biting animal

Species of animals	Frequency	Percent
Cattle	3	0.9%
Dog	300	95%
Donkey	5	1.6%
Wild animals	1	0.3%
Horse	1	0.3%
Man	6	1.9%
Total	316	100%

5.5. Status of dogs involved in the bite:

Of the 316 respondents, a majority (94.3%) of the victims mentioned that the disease (rabies) status of the dogs involved in the bite incidents was rabid, 5.7% victims mentioned that the biting dogs were normal (Table3)(from the suspected dog bites based on criteria published by Tepsumethanon *et al.,* 2005(if the dog is >1 month or not known, sick less than 10 days or not known, gradual onset of illness or not known, symptoms and signs progressing or not known ,no sign of circling or not known, showed at least 2 of the 17 following signs or symptoms during the last week of life: drooping jaw, abnormal sound in barking, dry drooping tongue, licking its own urine, abnormal licking of water, regurgitation, altered behavior, biting and eating abnormal objects, aggression, biting with no provocation, running without apparent reason, stiffness upon running or walking, restlessness, bites during quarantine, appearing sleepy,) imbalance of gait, frequent demonstration of the "dog sitting" position) (Tepsumethanon *et al.,* 2005).

Table 3: status of biting animals, on the basis of descriptive case histories 94.3% of animals that caused bite injuries were classified as suspected rabid (298).The status of animals that bit the remaining 18(5.7 %) of cases visited was normal.

	Frequency	Percent (%)
Not rabid	18	5.7%
Rabid	298	94.3%
Total	316	100%

5.6. Ownership of biting animals:

The study shows victims were predominantly bitten by neighbor dogs (108/316; 34.2%), rather than by owned dogs (101/316; 32.0%) (Figure 3).Of the316 bite victims, 74/316(23.4%) and 33 /316(10.4%) cases were bitten by a stray dog and known but far dogs respectively.

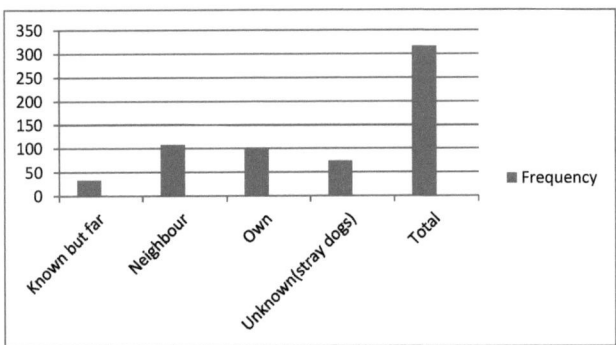

Figure 3: Ownership of biting animal

5.7. Anatomical site of bite

This study shows that most common bitten part of the body was legs (67.4%). Most (91.7%) bites victims were inflicted on the extremities with 67.4% on the legs, 21.5% on the arms/hand and 2.8% on the arms /legs, and 4.1% bite were on trunk.

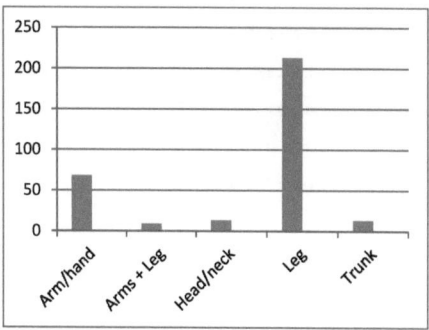

Figure 4: Illustrates the anatomic location of dog bite wounds of the victim.

5.8. Severity of bite

Study shows that out of 316 bite victims 35.8% were category i, 42.7% were category ii and 21.5% were category iii according to WHO classification(i) touching or feeding animals, licks on skin, ii(nibbling of uncovered skin ,minor scratches or abrasion without bleeding and iii (single or multiple transdermal bites)

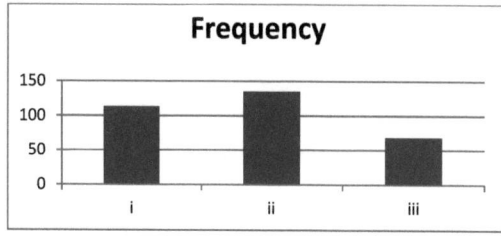

Figure 5: shows wound severity

5.9. Rabies post exposure prophylaxis and wound management

For those who visited the health center, 38% of them received rabies vaccine, 15.8% received both rabies vaccine and tetanus vaccine and 1% of bite victim received only tetanus vaccine. Among those who did not completed post exposure prophylaxis, 4.7 % stated wound had healed, 0.6% stated as they didn't believe that PEP cures and 0.6% shifted to traditional (Table 4). Of 316 responses to questions regarding wound washing, 3.8% reported washing the wound with soap prior to presentation at the health centre; The use of soap in washing animal bite wounds as a means of inactivating virus at the bite site is a recommendation of WHO (1992). Out of 170 cases started rabies vaccine, 123(72.2%) completed rabies vaccine. In addition, 51 of 316 (16.1%) patients received tetanus toxoid and 12/316(3.8%) washed wound by water and soap

Table 4: Rabies post exposure prophylaxis and other practices

	Frequency	Percent
unspecified	93	29.4%
Don't know extent of treatment	10	3.2%
No(only advice)	27	8.5%
Rabies vaccine	120	38.0%
Rabies vaccine and tetanus vaccine	50	15.8%
Tetanus vaccine	1	0.3%
Wound washing with water and soap	12	3.8%
Total	316	100.0%

5.10. Severity and anatomic locations of bite wounds

There was no a significant difference between the severity and anatomic locations of bite wounds Majority of bite on leg, head and arm/hand was class ii while on the trunk wound class iii was recorded.

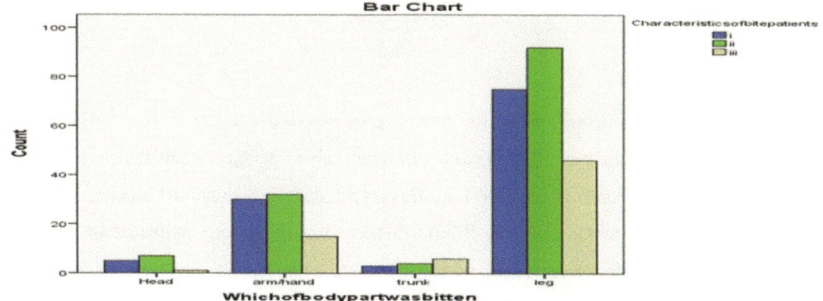

Figure 6. Comparision of age class and body part bitten showed in all age class characteristic of bite (severity of wound) on leg was class iii.

5.11. Distribution of bite injuries on the body according to age group of dog bite patients

Patients with injuries to the head/ neck, arm/hand, leg and trunk were predominantly younger When comparing with the total study population (Table 5).

Table 5: Distribution of bite injuries on the body according to age group

		Which of body part was bitten				Total
		Arm/hand	Head/neck	Leg	Trunk	
age	1(1-19)	40	7	120	8	175
	2(20-29	17	3	41	1	62
	3(30-50	11	2	37	1	51
	4(>50)	9	1	15	3	28
Total		77	13	213	13	316

6. DISCUSSION:

Ethiopia has been considered among the most rabies affected country in the world with an estimated annual occurrence of 10, 000 cases of human rabies which is equivalent to 18.6 cases per 100, 000 peoples (Fiqadu *et al.*, 1997). In the present study a high annual incidence of about 137/100, 000 was determined in Lemu-Bilbilo district. The incidences estimated in this study were based on only bite victim cases of the diseases. This annual incidence of bites from suspected rabid animals was derived from 316 people bitten by a suspected animal within 12 months.

The breeding season of dogs may cause the seasonal difference in dog bite prevalence in many countries. In Ethiopia the breeding season for dogs is August to October. In this study the incidences of bites were found higher in summer and autumn months. This is in line with the findings of Hanna and Selby, (1996) that they estimated that the highest incidence of bites occurred during the summer months. It is during these months that dogs are breeding and hence male dogs in a group are following a bitch for mating. Provocative actions and interference made by people especially children during this time might be contributing for higher bite(Hanna and Selby, 1996).

The risk factors for human dog bites identified in this study are very similar to those of other studies conducted elsewhere, (Overall and Love, 2001). This study found that males were statistically more likely to have experienced dog bites than female participants. This has been presented in a number of epidemiological studies on dog bite characteristics (Rosado *et al.*, 2009; Yalcin *et al.*, 2012). This can also be related to boys being more likely to display risk behavior, as shown in this study. For instance, dog bite injuries were more common in children, particularly those aged 1–19.9 years, and dog bite injuries to the lower extremities were more common (67.4%) than to other body parts, irrespective of the age of the victim in this study. This result is in contrast to some other studies in which more bite injuries were reported to the head, neck and face (Daniels *et al.*, 2008). Dog bites more common in males than females .The incidence of dog bite was recorded in all age groups but was elevated in age groups of 0-19 year and males were the primary victims. Males are affected more often than the females, as they constituted the working majority who were actively engaged in outdoor activities. These findings corroborate similar observations from other study (Singh et al., 2001).It has also been suggested that bites in children are more likely to be reported than in adults because more parental concern towards children or the severity of their injuries (Sacks et al., 1996).

Majority of children was bitten on leg. When we compare still children under 19.9 was predominantly bitten on head/neck, trunk and arm/hand. Almost one half of all dog bites involve an animal owned by the victim's family or neighbours. Most dog bites are inflicted by a known owned dog, at or near the dog's home which agree with other study (Sacks et al. 1996).A large percentage of dog bite victims are children in the developed world, pet dogs (owned dogs or neighbors' dogs) which are known to the victim are most commonly involved in bite incidents to the head, neck and face. This may be due to the short height of children and playful relations with pets; kissing, hugging and petting (Sacks et al., 1996). It is also likely that the victims (children) would have used a hand or leg to abuse/ tease the dogs or to separate fighting dogs or defending dog attacks, resulting in more bites on the extremities (Rosado et al .,2009). Rabid dog bites to the upper body and extremities (head, neck, arm, hand) are more dangerous than bites to the lower extremities.

Among bites by various animals, dog bites being the major cause of injury to humans is supported by previous findings in many parts of the world, particularly Africa and Asia. Domestic dogs are the principal reservoirs and vectors of rabies (WHO, 2001; Tang et al., 2005). The study showed that animal bites are still a major problem in this area of Ethiopia and confirms previous surveys indicating that they are also common in many parts of the country. In several studies, dogs were the primary animal Species implicated, accounting for 63–80% of cases (Yimer et al., 2002; Deresa et al., 2010). In the current study, dog bites contributed to 95% of cases needing rabies post-exposure prophylaxis. This is in agreement with previous studies conducted in Ethiopia (Yimer et al., 2002; Deresa et al., 2010) and India (Ichhpujani et al., 2008). The most common anatomical location of bites was the leg (67.4%), which was also reported in other studies (Ichhpujani et al., 2008; Dwyer et al 2007). The second anatomical locations in frequency were the arms and hands; we did not notice significant differences between the reported severity of bite and its location.

Children constituted the highest proportion of human cases reported for treatment of injuries caused by bites of rabies-suspected animals, mainly domestic dogs. Understanding the dynamics of rabies in domestic dogs is needed to facilitate the designing of more effective control measures that could reduce deaths from the disease, of which >95% result from bites by domestic dogs (Tang *et al.*, 2005).

Understanding people's level of knowledge about dog bites and the risk of potential zoonotic disease transmission particularly rabies is important for planning an awareness education program. To prevent human rabies, rapid intervention following a dog bite incident, consisting of appropriate wound management and administration of post exposure vaccination where indicated is important. Also critical is an efficient and effective surveillance systems that detect cases in humans and animals and adopting an integrated approach in the management of the disease prevention and control strategies. On the contrary, only (3.8%) victims reportedly did wash their wound with soap and water at home before visiting the hospital for medical treatment. Cleaning and flushing of the bite wound with soap and water immediately after being bitten is one of the most important steps recommended by the WHO (WHO, 1996; WHO, 2010) is required.

The use of traditional treatment by 34.8% of respondents shows high reliance on this unproven medication. Deresa *et al.*, 2010 and his colleagues noted that most fatal human rabies cases recoded in Ethiopia were mostly helped exhaustively by traditional healers. So much has to be done to reduce the high reliance of victims on traditional treatment by raising their awareness and increasing availability of post exposure anti-rabies vaccines. There are preliminary reports of anti-rabies activities of some commonly used herbs in the traditional anti-rabies treatment practice in Ethiopia. Clearly, there is need for increased vaccination coverage of dogs to reduce rabies transmission among the susceptible animals and humans. Dog vaccination campaigns would even be more successful when accompanied with accessible and affordable PEP for humans. participation; however, with appropriate efforts, these can all be addressed(Deresa *et al.*, 2010).

7. CONCLUSION AND RECOMMENDATIONS

Rabies is a fatal neurologic illness transmitted to people by direct contact with the saliva of a rabid animal, normally through a bite. Animal bites continue to be a problem in Ethiopia. As a result, there are many people at risk of rabies virus infection. Among bites by various animals, dog bites being the major cause of injury to humans. The incidence of dog bites was greater amongst children and greater in males than females across all age groups, and lack of sufficient awareness about the disease and high reliance on traditional treatment that interfere with timely post exposure management.

In light of above conclusion; the following points are recommended:-

- Public education must be an integral part of the efforts to decrease the incidence of animal bites and to ensure that they are managed properly.
- In addition to the currently recommended strategy of controlling the dog population, and of vaccinating domesticated animals, a better surveillance for dog rabies by appropriate laboratory investigations of suspected animals is also recommended.
- Intervention measures should include public educational programs on dog behavior, dog-child interaction, the risk of dog bites and bite wound management (e.g., washing with soap and water), particularly for children
- The public health implications of animal attacks are significant, and awareness of the risks to young children needs to be emphasized.

8. REFERENCES

Bogel, K., and Motschwiller, E. (1986) Incidence of rabies and post exposure treatment in developing countries. *B. World Health Organ.* **64**: 883–887.

Bogel, K.and Meslin. F. (1990): Economics of human and canine rabies elimination: Guidelines for programme orientation. *Bull. World Health Organ.*, **68**:281-91.

Central statistic Authority, CSA) (2014): Federal Democratic Republic of Ethiopia, Population Projection of Ethiopia for All Regions at Wereda Level from 2014 – 2017

Cleaveland, S., Kaare, M. ,Tiringa, P., Mlengeya, T.and Barrat, J. (2003): A dog rabies vaccination campaign in rural Africa: Impact of the incidence of dog rabies and human dog-bite injuries. Vaccine. **21**:1965-73

Cleaveland.S., Fever, E.M. Kaare, M.and Coleman, P.G. (2002): Estimating human rabies mortality in the United Republic of Tanzania from dog bite injuries. *Bull. World Health Organ.* . 80:304-10.

Daniels, D., Ritzi, R., O'Neil, J.and Scherer, L (2008) Analysis of nonfatal dog bites in children. *J. Trauma Inj. Infect. Critical Care* , **66**: 17–22.

Deressa, A., Ali, A. Beyene, M.. Newaye, S. and Yimer, E. (2010): The status of rabies in Ethiopia: A retrospective record review. *Ethiopian J. Health Manag.*, **24**: 127–132.

Dwyer, J.P., Douglas, T.S.,and van, A.B.(2007). Dog bites injuries in children – a review of data from a South African paediatric trauma unit. *S. Afr. Med. J.*, **97**: 597–600.

Fekadu, M. (1997): Human rabies surveillance and control in Ethiopia. In: proceeding of the southern and eastern African rabies group meeting 1997 March 4–6; Nairobi. Kenya

Hanna, T.L. and Selby, L.A.(1996). Characteristics of the human and pet populations in animal bite incidents recorded at two Air Force bases. *Public Health Rep.*, **96**, 6,580-584.

Humphrey, D. M. Fredros,O. O.. Eliningaya, J. K.and Ladslaus, L. M. (2010): Retrospective analysis of suspected rabies cases reported at Bugando Referral Hospital. Mwanza. Tanzania. *J. Infect. Dis.*, **2**: 216-220

Ichhpujani, R.L., Mala, C., Veena, M., Singh, J., Bhardwaj, M., Bhattacharya, D., *et al.*(2008): Epidemiology of animal bites and rabies cases in India. A multicentric study. *J. Commun. Dis.*, **40**: 27–36.

Jackson, A.C.and Wunner, W.H. (2007): Rabies. 2nd edition. San Diego: Academic press.

Knobel, D.L., Cleaveland, S., Coleman,P.G.. Fθvre, E.M.. Meltzer, M.I.and Miranda, M.E.. *et al.* (2005):Re-evaluating the burden of rabies in Africa and Asia. *Bull. World Health Organ.*, **83**:360-8.

Meslin,F. Fishbein, D.and Matter, H. (1994): Rationale and Prospects For Rabies Elimination In Developing Countries. In: Rupprecht CE. Dietzschold B. Koprowski H. editors. Lyssaviruses. Berlin: Springer Verlag;. pp. 1–26.

Overall, K. and Love, M. (2001) .Dog bites to humans–demography, epidemiology, injury and risk. *J.A.V.M.A.*, **218**: 1923–1934

Paulos, A, Eshetu, Y., Bethelhem, N., Abebe B, and Badeg, Z., et al. (2002) A study on the prevalence ofanimal rabies in Addis Ababa during 1999–2002:*Ethiopian Veterinary Journal* **7**: 69–77.

Rosado, B., Garcia-Belenguer, S., Leon, M.and Palacio, J. (2009): A comprehensive study of dog bites in Spain, 1995–2004. Vet J. **179**: 383–391.

Sacks, J.J., Kresnow, M., and Houston, B. (1996): Dog bites: how big a problem? Inj. Prev. 2: 52–54.3.

Singh, J., Jain, D.C., Bhatia, R., Ichhpujani, R.L., Harit, A.K. and Panda, R.C. (2001). Epidemiological characteristics of rabies in Delhi and surrounding areas 1998. *Indian Paediatrics,* **38**:1354-60.

Tang, X., Luo, M., Zhang, S. Fooks, A., Hu, R.and Tu, C. (2005): Pivotal role of dogs in rabies transmission. China. *Emerg. Infec.t Dis.*, **11**:1970-2. .

Tepsumethanon, V. Wilde,H. and Meslin,F.(2005):Six Criteria for Rabies Diagnosis in Living Dogs. *J. Med. Assoc. Thai,* **88**: 419-22

Warrell, D.A.and Warell,M.J. (1995): Human rabies: A continuing challenge in the tropical world. *Schweiz Med Wochenschr.* **125**:879–885.

World Health Organization (1987): Guidelines for Dog Rabies Control. World Health Organization. Geneva (VPH/83.43).

World Health Organization (1998): World survey of rabies no. 32 for the year 1996. Geneva: The Organization;Pp 1-27

World health organization (2001): Strategies for the control and elimination of rabies in Asia. Geneva: The World Health Organis. Department of Communicable Disease Surveillance and Response.

World Health Organization (2010): Rabies vaccines: WHO position paper.*Wkly epidemiol. Rec.*, **85**: 309–320.

Yalcin, E., Kentsu, H.and Batmaz, H. (2012). A survey of animal bites on humans in Bursa, Turkey. *J. Vet. Behaviour,* **7**: 233–237.

Yimer, E., Neway, B., Girma, T., Mekonnen, Y., Yoseph, B., Badeg, Z., *et al.* (2002). Situation of rabies in Ethiopia: a retrospective study 1990–2000. *J. Health Dev.*, **16**: 105–112.

YOUR KNOWLEDGE HAS VALUE

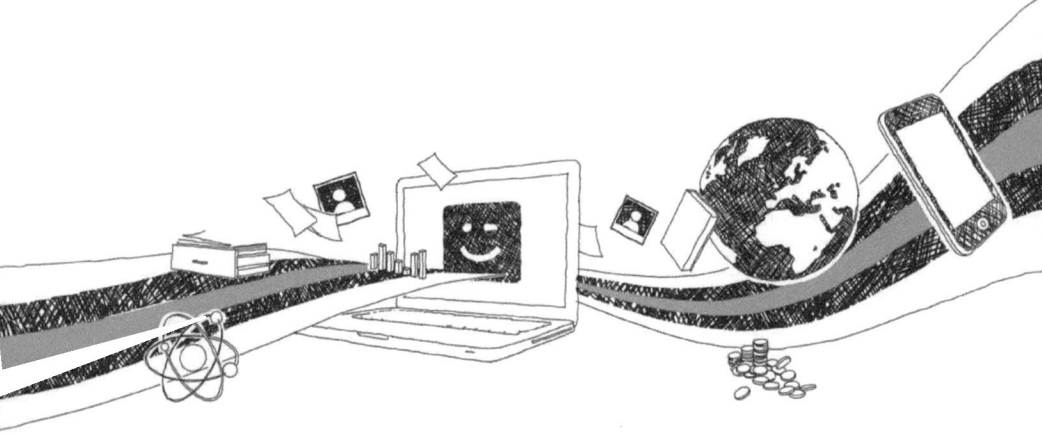

- We will publish your bachelor's and master's thesis, essays and papers

- Your own eBook and book - sold worldwide in all relevant shops

- Earn money with each sale

Upload your text at www.GRIN.com and publish for free

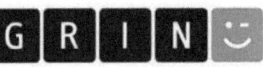